THE LITTLE BOOK OF
POOP

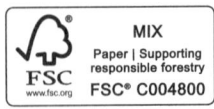

Published in 2024 by OH!
An Imprint of Welbeck Non-Fiction Limited,
part of Welbeck Publishing Group.
Offices in: London – 20 Mortimer Street, London W1T 3JW
and Sydney – Level 17, 207 Kent St, Sydney NSW 2000 Australia
www.welbeckpublishing.com

Compilation text © Welbeck Non-Fiction Limited 2024
Design © Welbeck Non-Fiction Limited 2024

Disclaimer:
All trademarks, copyright, quotations, company names, registered names, products, characters, logos and catchphrases used or cited in this book are the property of their respective owners. This book is a publication of *OH! An imprint of Welbeck Publishing Group Limited* and has not been licensed, approved, sponsored, or endorsed by any person or entity.

All rights reserved. No part of this publication may be reproduced, stored in a retrieval system, or transmitted in any form or by any means (including electronic, mechanical, photocopying, recording, or otherwise) without prior written permission from the publisher.

ISBN 978-1-80069-624-2

Compiled and written by: Malcolm Croft
Editorial: Victoria Denne
Design: Stephen Cary
Project manager: Russell Porter
Production: Marion Storz

A CIP catalogue record for this book is available from the British Library

Printed in Dubai

10 9 8 7 6 5 4 3 2 1

THE LITTLE BOOK OF
POOP

STINKY WIT AND WISDOM

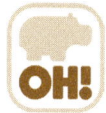

CONTENTS

INTRODUCTION – 6

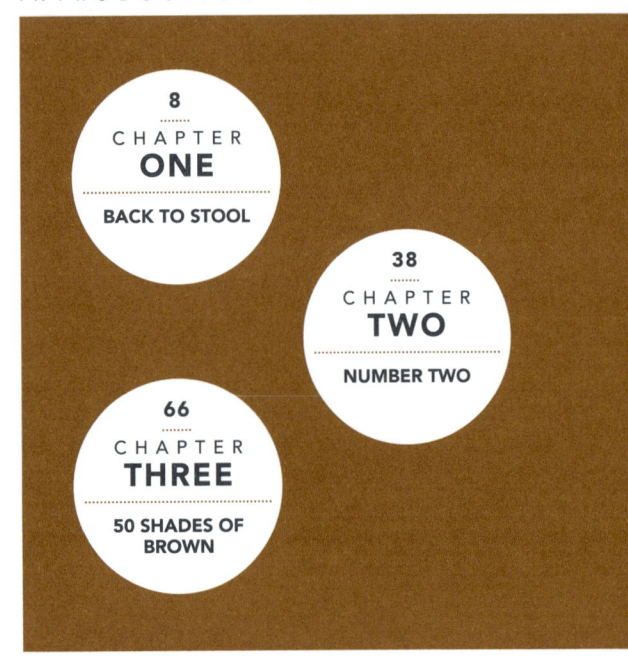

8
CHAPTER
ONE
BACK TO STOOL

38
CHAPTER
TWO
NUMBER TWO

66
CHAPTER
THREE
50 SHADES OF BROWN

96
CHAPTER
FOUR

BOTTOMS UP!

126
CHAPTER
FIVE

IT HAPPENS

152
CHAPTER
SIX

WIPE OUT

INTRODUCTION

Welcome aboard the world's first portable *poopepedia*! (I bet that's a sentence you probably never thought you'd read.)

As perfectly formed as this tiny tome feels in your hands – it's the same length as a perfect stool, FYI – this meandering sojourn down the u-bend will by no means be smooth sailing. No, this is going to be a hard and lumpy float down into the darkest bowels and anals – sorry, *annals* of history, to showcase the very best of poop, glorious poop – humankind's oldest and greatest obsession and guilty pleasure.

Thankfully, this little book is up to the job: it's completely full of shit. 100 per cent crap. As polished as a turd can be. Without wanting to fart in our own trumpet, this *Little Book of Poop* is perfect for the nincompoopers, turd-nerds and stool-gazers who love nothing more than to curl one off and gaze in awe at their creation. If that's you, pull up a toilet seat and drop anchor. You're home.

Published to celebrate the 540 millionth anniversary of the very first butthole – thanks, sea sponges, you're the best – *The Little Book of Poop* is as essential as it is easily digestible. Poop isn't just shits and giggles, after all; it's important, too. Poop defines us. It sticks us all together. We are birthed in poop, and we die in diapers as our soul flushes away to the great toilet in the sky. Every single day between those two events, shit happens. (Sometimes twice if you eat a lot of fibre.) Without poop, what are we? Just a bag of skin and bones.

Crammed with all the butt-based buffoonery you need without ever feeling bloated or constipated, this little guide lifts the lid on poop's many shapes, sizes and backstories. And the only straining you'll be doing is bending over backwards with laughter.

Yes, this is perfect toilet humour for the next time you need to bake a loaf by the pool. Enjoy!

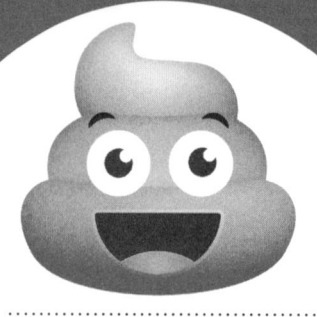

CHAPTER
ONE

BACK TO STOOL

To celebrate the fact that poop comes in all shapes and sizes (and smells), this compacted – sorry, *compact* compendium of coprology is constipated with a feast of feces so flushed with facts that you'll feel delightfully full of knowledge come the final sheet of paper.

It's time to learn the glory of poop. It's time to go back to stool…

BACK TO STOOL

WHAT'S BROWN AND STICKY?

A stick!

POOPHORIA

That good, good feeling of having pooped a poop so perfect you stare at it proudly.

BACK TO STOOL

> **Just poopin'. You know how I be.**

Michael Scott, *The Office (U.S.)*,
Season 6, Episode 10, 2009.

You can't polish a turd… but you can roll it in glitter!

The perfect poop size is ideally between four and eight inches long.

96

The number of bags of (non-alien) poop on the moon's surface left by twelve U.S. astronauts.

Neil Armstrong, the first man to walk on the moon, left four bags of poop* when he moonwalked in 1969. He was there for just 21 hours and 36 minutes.

* To be fair, who wouldn't be shitting themselves?

BACK TO STOOL

Once a week, sloths descend to the trunk of their trees, stand on their hind legs and shake their bodies until poop falls out. It's called the poop dance.

> # Well, I sure feel bad for whoever finds my bag.

Buzz Aldrin, in a tweet, when asked about the U.S.'s return to the moon in the next decade.

* FYI, Aldrin was the first human to go to the toilet on the moon.

BACK TO STOOL

In France, stepping on dog poop with your left foot is considered good luck.*

* You're shit out of luck if it ends up on your right foot.

If something looks like shit and smells like shit – it's probably shit.

BACK TO STOOL

SCATOLOGY *

The term used to describe the academic study of poop.

* Don't confuse this with eschatology, the study of the end of the world. Or scatting, a type of nonsense-syllable singing heard in jazz music.

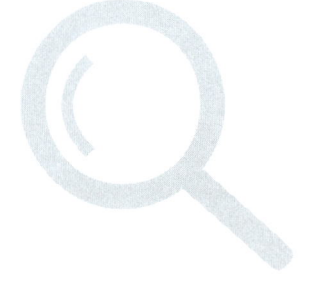

POOP PHOBIAS

Coprophobia – the fear of poop

Acrorectophobia – the fear of buttholes

Pugophobia – the fear of buttocks

Trypophobia – the fear of holes

Osmophobia – the fear of smells

Mysophobia – the fear of germs

Kastanophobia – the fear of the colour brown

BACK TO STOOL

NINCOMPOOP

An English word to describe a silly or foolish person. Dates back to the 1670s.

In 2016, NASA sponsored the "Space Poop Challenge" to see if contestants could design an improved spacesuit toilet system that could be worn for more than 144 hours.

The contest was won by Dr Thatcher Cardon who invented a "perineal access port", which we won't go into here…

BACK TO STOOL

STEATORRHEA

A floater so thick
with fatty foods that
it won't flush.

7

The average number of sheets used per average butt per average wipe.

BACK TO STOOL

1592

The year the first flush toilet was invented by Sir John Harington, godson of Elizabeth I. He built one for himself and one for the queen. It was called Ajax.

Alas, his invention was ignored – for two hundred years – until Alexander Cummings developed a similar design in 1775.

> # Must eat, then poop, then eat some more, then eat while pooping.

Homer Simpson, *The Simpsons*, Season 18, Episode 4, 2006.

BACK TO STOOL

In the 1890s, New York suffered from a manure crisis that would be unthinkable today. More than 100,000 horses were pooping 2,500,000 lbs on the streets every day!

The emergency was debated at the world's first international urban planning conference in New York in 1898, but no solution was found… until 1900, when the first automobiles became available.

PARCOPRESIS

The term used to describe the fear of pooping in public toilets, otherwise known as psychogenic fecal retention, or shy bowel syndrome.

BACK TO STOOL

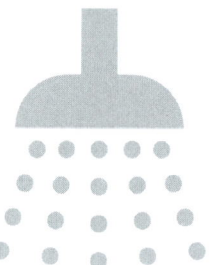

ONE IN TEN

The number of Americans who have admitted, to the Huffington Post at least, that they poop in the shower.

Are you the one?

POOP-SOCKING

The term used to describe someone so engrossed in playing a video game that they won't pause to go poop. So, they put a sock in it.

> **I would probably eat shit if someone told me, 'If you eat this bowl of poop every single day, you'll look younger.'**

Kim Kardashian in an interview with *Allure* magazaine, 2022.

25.6 IN (67.5 CM)

The length of the world's largest (dinosaur) poop, discovered in Buffalo, Harding County, South Dakota, USA, in 2020.

The poop is the largest coprolite (fossilized poop) found on Earth so far. It weighs 20.47 lbs (9.28 kg) and is thought to be around 70 million years old. The coprolite was given the nickname "Barnum" after Barnum Brown, the paleontologist who discovered the first *Tyrannosaurus rex*.

BACK TO STOOL

1853

The year that the first flushable toilet was installed in the White House, Washington D.C. The rather aptly named Millard Millmore was president at the time.

> **It's enough to poop every other day. That will be better for the whole world.***

Jair Bolsonaro, 2019.

* These are the comments made by the controversial right-wing President after Brazil's deforestation and agriculture were blamed for a quarter of the planet's greenhouse effect.

POONAMI

The term to describe a baby's poop explosion, or an adult's after one too many coffees. A tsunami of poop!

11,023,100,000,000 lbs.*

The amount of animal poop that, by 2030, will be generated by all the world's billions of livestock each year.

* Five billion tons!

CHAPTER TWO

NUMBER TWO

It's time to poop or get off the pot! Welcome to round two – the second push, always the hardest. But don't worry, we've got you covered. All you've got to do is pull up a pew and let it all hang loose.

From historical dates to skidmark-stained stats and everything in between, this chapter is a smorgasbord of shit where no factoid is left to float alone. Lock the door, and let's get down to business…

NUMBER TWO

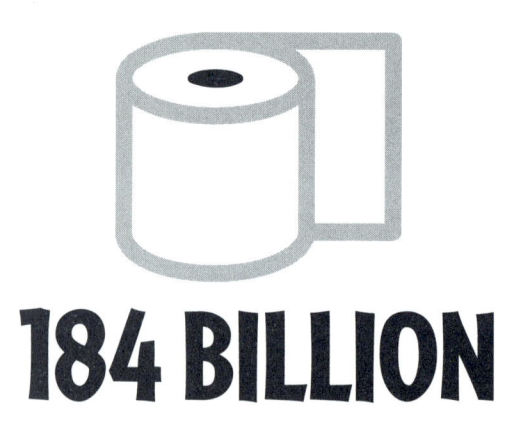

184 BILLION

The number of toilet rolls flushed away every year worldwide.*

* A single pine tree produces 1,500 rolls of toilet paper.

Bristol Stool Scale

According to the Bristol Stool Scale, the world's number-one guide to number twos, poop comes in distinct shapes and sizes.

1. Separate hard lumps – indicates severe constipation.

2. Sausage-shaped, but lumpy – indicates constipation.

3. Like a sausage, but with cracks on its surface – normal.

4. Like a snake, smooth and soft – normal.

5. Soft blobs with clear-cut edges – lacks fibre.

6. Fluffy pieces with ragged edges, a bit mushy – mild diarrhoea.

7. Watery, no solid pieces, entirely liquid – severe diarrhoea.

NUMBER TWO

WHAT'S THE WORST FEELING IN THE WORLD?

A fart with a lump in it.*

* Commonly known as a "shart".

STERCOBILIN

The chemical to blame for making your poop that dirty brown colour.

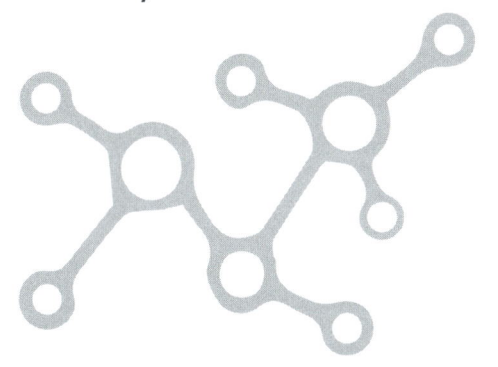

NUMBER TWO

> Let me assure you that there is nothing funny about going up to a nice, clean, unsuspecting urinal, dropping your pants, then turning around… squatting over that urinal… maybe pulling your butt cheeks apart with your hands, and then laying out a big fudge dragon for all the world to see!

Mr Mackey
South Park, Season 10, Episode 9, 2006.

> I'm horrible to live with. I don't clean. My clothes end up wherever I take them off. I forget to flush the toilet. Friends will tell me, 'Megan, you totally pinched a loaf in my toilet and didn't flush.'

Megan Fox in an interview with *FHM* magazine, 2007.

GONGFERMERS

The name given to medieval laborers who shovelled and transported poop away from the privy pits of private houses. They were paid handsomely to do so.

> # My Lord, I had forgot the fart.

Queen Elizabeth, welcoming home Edward de Vere, 17th Earl of Oxford, in 1700. The Earl had farted in the presence of the queen and was so ashamed he left the country – for seven years.

NUMBER TWO

> "The great thing about having a bunch of kids is that they just remind you that you're the person who takes them to go poop. That's who you are!"

Angelina Jolie, 2013.

> And thou shalt have a paddle upon thy weapon; and it shall be, when thou wilt ease thyself abroad, thou shalt dig therewith, and shalt turn back and cover that which cometh from thee.

Deuteronomy, 23:13

NUMBER TWO

50 per cent of Americans would prefer not to talk about pooping.

116 HOURS!

It was Jimmy De Frenne, a 48-year-old Belgian man, who, in 2019, decided to spend seven days (165 hours) straight sitting on the toilet. His legs gave out after 116 hours.

Still, a world record. It's unknown how much pooping occurred.

NUMBER TWO

According to the *Guinness Book of World Records*, Canada is the nation most in love with the poop emoji. It accounts for 0.48 per cent of all emojis posted by Canadians. The Australians, Americans and British are the runners-up.

* The Pile of Poo emoji in Unicode is U+1F4A9.

💩

According to Statista, more than 40,000 Americans hurt themselves in "toilet-seat related accidents" every year.

NUMBER TWO

Toilet Humour Playlist: Songs to Poop to

American toilets flush in the key of E-flat.

To celebrate this fact, here are our top ten favourite songs originally recorded in that key. Now you can flush along with the classics!

1. "Sweet Child O' Mine" – Guns N' Roses
2. "Jailhouse Rock" – Elvis Presley
3. "All Along the Watchtower" – Jimi Hendrix

4. "I Want to Know What Love Is" – Foreigner
5. "Every Breath You Take" – The Police
6. "Beat It" – Michael Jackson
7. "More Than Words" – Extreme
8. "The Man Who Sold the World" – Nirvana
9. "I Miss You" – Blink-182
10. "Simple Man" – Lynyrd Skynyrd

NUMBER TWO

25 October, 1760

On this day, English King George II died on the toilet.

He had just finished his morning cup of hot chocolate.*

* Not a poophemism.

34 BILLION

The number of gallons that wastewater treatment facilities in the United States process every single day.

* It would take 32 billion days to fill up the Grand Canyon's 1.1 trillion gallons worth of land.

NUMBER TWO

STOOL-GAZING

The term used to describe that glance down the bowl at your poop after pooping. We all do it. If it's a good clean poop, the feeling of pride you fill is called *shatisfaction*.

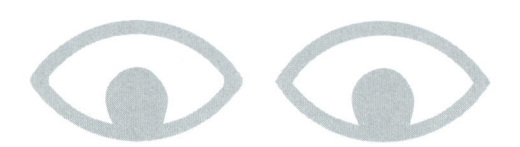

> Why do I always meet women as I'm leaving the dog park with a big bag of poop? And it's always on the day I forgot my dog.

Dana Gould

NUMBER TWO

> **Monica:** He pooped in my shoe.
>
> **Phoebe:** Which one?
>
> **Monica:** Those cute little black ones I wear all the time.
>
> **Phoebe**: No, which one? The right or left? 'Cause the left one is lucky.

Friends, Season 1, Episode 19, 1995.

> I was driving and heavy breathing, because I'm about to have a butt baby. I let a little water out of my levees, like a Hershey's Kiss that's been sitting in the sun too long. I hovered over my steering wheel for leverage, and my body was like, 'NO, WE WANT IT ALL.' I just filled my underwear with a travel-size pillow worth of brisket. Then I waddled inside, took a shower and had a four-hour shame nap.

Nick Kroll, 2016.

NUMBER TWO

> **"**
> It was the ultimate, giant, chocolate mess.
> **"**

Julie Moss, legendary Ironman triathlete, lost control of her bowels during the Hawaii Ironman in 1982.

GASTROCOLIC REFLEX

The scientific term to describe that powerful urge to poop after that first cup of morning coffee.

NUMBER TWO

Gut Microbiome

Gut health is all the rage these days and for good reason too – a healthy gut means happy poop. These are the top 15 foods to poop like a champ.

1. Nuts
2. Prunes
3. Kiwis
4. Flaxseeds
5. Pears
6. Beans
7. Rhubarb
8. Artichokes
9. Kefir
10. Figs
11. Sweet potatoes
12. Lentils
13. Chia seeds
14. Avocados
15. Oat bran

High Fibre

Fibre helps you poop straight. Become fibre's friend:

Soluble fibre

Oat bran, barley, nuts, seeds, beans, lentils and peas absorb water. Softens your stool and reduces the risk of heart disease.

Insoluble fibre

Wheat bran, vegetables and whole grains. Adds bulk to poop for better passing.

CHAPTER THREE

50 SHADES OF BROWN

From birth to death, and every day in between, humanity is swamped with poop. It becomes us. From health to wealth, mind to matter and soul to hole, our fascination with all things sticky and brown is as normal as taking the dog for a walk.

So, let's get the party pooping started, and embrace feces with two hands* as this chapter dares us to do daily with a wealth of turd-based trivia.

* Not literally of course. Use a pooper-scooper.

50 SHADES OF BROWN

DEFECATION

The polite word for the act of pooping, and origin of the word feces, comes from the Latin phrase *de faece*, meaning "from dregs".

92

The number of days an average person will spend on the toilet in their lifetime – roughly one-third of a year.

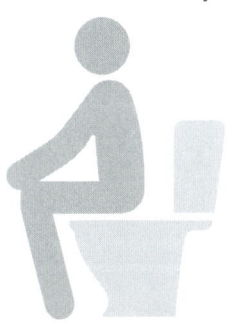

50 SHADES OF BROWN

11,000

The total amount, in U.S. dollars, the average American spends on toilet paper* in their lifetime.

That's around 85 rolls, 13,000 sheets and approx. $180 a year.

Your butt's worth it.

* 384 trees, on average, are used to make enough toilet paper for one person to use within their lifetime.

1.2 MILLION MILES*

The total length of America's sewers. That's the equivalent distance of travelling to the moon and back. Twice.

*1,931,208 km!

According to the Dog Advisory Board, in 2023, Seattle was named the Dog Poop Capital of the United States.

San Francisco, Pittsburgh and Denver were not far behind.

47%

The percentage of American men whose beards are home to *enterococcus*, a bacteria found in poop. No judgement here. Well, some.

MINIMAL TURING TEST

In 2023, the "Minimal Turing Test" was devised as a psychology experiment to see what words are more human than others in a supposed test against AI machines.

More than 1,000 participants gave words for judges to guess whether they were given by humans or created by machines.

The judges concluded that "poop" was the one word most likely to convince a human being that you are not a robot.

> I had massive diarrhoea in my Rent-A-Car. I didn't just shit my pants; I shit my car. I was in a total state of shock. I finally got to the front desk of the hotel, almost in tears, and I said, 'My name is Jon Benjamin, I'm staying at this hotel, I had diarrhoea in my pants for the last two hours. Please help me. Just, please get me to the room.' Luckily, they were nice about it all.

H. Jon Benjamin, 2011.

DYSCHEZIA

The technical term for difficulty passing poop, usually from straining, pain or obstruction.

18%

A 2023 survey revealed that almost one-fifth of employees are so afraid to poop at work that they return home to do their business there. Another one-fifth simply hold the poop in all day.

* Another one-fifth of employees admit to pooping on another floor in the office.

30%

The percentage, according to Healthline, of American men who admit they wait up to three months before daring to poop at a new partner's home.

The American West has "more normal" poops than the American South.

50 SHADES OF BROWN

> # I'm going to the bathroom to read.*

Elvis Presley's last words, shortly before he died trying to poop on the toilet.

* Presley died because of his poor diet and constipation. He had a four-month-old compacted stool in his bowel. The strain of pooping caused Presley to have a heart attack.

Death on the Toilet

Persons of note who died upon their thrones…

1. Coolio, rapper
2. Elvis Presley, singer
3. Judy Garland, actor
4. George II, King of England
5. Lenny Bruce, comedian
6. Lupe Vélez, actor
7. Louis Kahn, architect
8. Don Simpson, movie producer
9. Evelyn Waugh, author
10. Catherine the Great, Empress of Russia

* As if dying isn't bad enough, humans poop themselves moments after death as a result of bowel and bladder muscles relaxing. So, dying on the toilet isn't such a bad thing.

50 SHADES OF BROWN

POOP DECK

A nautical term to describe the cabin at the rear of a ship where a captain navigates.

* If the poop deck is swamped by a high wave, it is said to be "pooped", the origin of the expression meaning "awash with exhaustion".

The word "poop" originated from the Latin *puppis*, meaning the back end, or stern, of a ship.

50 SHADES OF BROWN

To honour the seafaring history of the word "poop", here are our favourite naval poophemisms:

1. Drop anchor
2. A shot across the bowl
3. At loggerheads
4. Batten down the hatches
5. Chock a block
6. Copper bottomed
7. Dead in the water
8. Foul up
9. Give a wide berth
10. Hulking (something large and awkward)
11. Let the cat out of the bag
12. Logbook
13. Long haul
14. Loose cannon
15. Pipe down
16. Push the boat out
17. Running a tight ship
18. Scraping the barrel
19. Scuttlebutt
20. Shake a leg
21. Shiver me timbers
22. Slush fund
23. Three sheets to the wind
24. Touch and go
25. Walk the plank

> **The set smelled really sweet – delicious, really, like confectionary. You could have licked the chocolate right off the bowl.**

Danny Boyle, on the "Worst Toilet in Scotland" scene in 1996's *Trainspotting*. Different types of chocolates were used for the copious volumes of poop.

50 SHADES OF BROWN

> # Guys like you don't die on toilets.

Riggs (Mel Gibson) to Murtaugh (Danny Glover), who was pooping when he discovered a bomb in his toilet, *Lethal Weapon*, 1989.

COPROPHAGIA

The term to describe the eating of feces. Autocoprophagy is the eating of one's own poop.

50 SHADES OF BROWN

> **"**
> We're going to start by showing you the toilet and it's only going to get worse.*
> **"**

Joseph Stefano, screenwriter of *Psycho*, including the bathroom scene, a direct rebuke of the Hays Code, 1990.

* The first ever film to show a flushing toilet, or even a toilet on screen, was Alfred Hitchcock's 1960 masterpiece *Psycho*.

SAME DAY, DIFFERENT SHIT.

Poop Playlist: Handwashing Songs

Forget "Happy Birthday"! Wash your poop-covered hands to these songs. The choruses all last the desired hand-washing time – 20 seconds.

1. "I Want It That Way" – Backstreet Boys
2. "Love Shack" – The B-52's
3. "No Scrubs" – TLC
4. "So Fresh, So Clean" – OutKast
5. "Shake It Off" – Taylor Swift
6. "Thriller" Michael Jackson
7. "Let It Go" – Idina Menzel
8. "Ironic" – Alanis Morissette
9. "I'm Still Standing" – Elton John
10. "Oops... I Did It Again" – Britney Spears

$9.5 BILLION

The value, estimated in a U.N. report, that human waste would have if converted to biofuel.

50 SHADES OF BROWN

When a rectum is full of poop, stretch receptors in the wall of the anus are activated.

These receptors send signals via nerves to the cerebrum (a part of your brain).

The brain then tells you it's time to dump out.

> One thing we have to know before we really go any further: how do you feel about talking poop?*

Trey Parker, to Comedy Central Executives, before signing on with the channel to broadcast *South Park*, 2003.

* Mr Hankey, the show's infamous sentient poop character, was created by Parker's father while he was toilet-training Trey to encourage his son to flush his poop. If he did not, "Mr Hankey" would come to life and kill him.

50 SHADES OF BROWN

According to the Centers for Disease Control and Prevention, approx. one trillion germs can live in one gram* of poop.

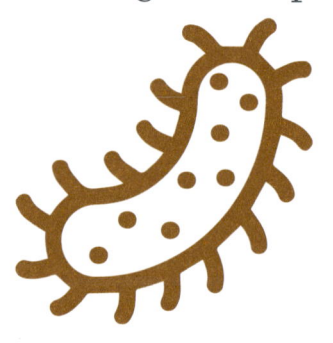

* Roughly the weight of a paper clip.

The average American male drops about 150 grams (about one-third of a pound) of poop every day. That's the equivalent of five tons in a lifetime!

CHAPTER
FOUR

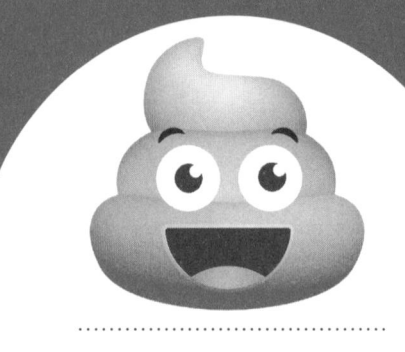

BOTTOMS UP

When it comes to poop, every hole's a goal. From the food we eat to the shit we sniff, poop is a part of everyday life, not some dirty little secret best kept repressed.

This chapter dives deep into all that's perfect about poop, one nugget of knowledge at a time. Take your time and breathe in that perfectly baked loaf… it's the best thing you'll do all day.

BOTTOMS UP

The next time you host a party, remember this fun party fact:

Diarrhoea is classified into four categories:

1. Osmotic

2. Secretory

3. Exudative

4. Rapid intestinal transit

15

The average number of times a person farts a day.*

* We expel about 1,000 ml of farts per day; that's enough gas to fill a two-litre bottle of soda. (Not that you'd want to do that kind of thing.)

Common Fart Phrases

1. "Whoever smelt it, dealt it."
2. "Whoever denied it, supplied it."
3. "Whoever detected it, ejected it."
4. "The smeller's the fella!"
5. "Whoever rhymed it, crimed it."
6. "Whoever observed it, served it."

Which one do you say?

Pantone 448C

Regarded as the ugliest colour, Pootone – sorry, *Pantone* 448C, also known as opaque couché, is the colour most associated with poop.

BOTTOMS UP

97%

The number of American males (and 90 per cent of females) who don't meet the daily recommended amount of fibre.

> If you're really a mean person you're going to come back as a fly and eat poop.

Kurt Cobain, *Monk Magazine*, 1993.

ONE IN SIX

A recent survey revealed that 16 per cent of cellphones are contaminated with *E. coli*, the bacteria found in feces.

26,000 lbs

The amount the average American poops in their lifetime. That's the equivalent weight of a school bus!

BOTTOMS UP

The amount of poop produced by all humans on earth in one year is approx. 640 billion lbs (290 billion kg)*!

* That's 1.5 million tons a day!

> Poop humour is fun. If you do the toilet scenes well and commit to them, they can be powerful.

Sandra Bullock

BOTTOMS UP

> All right, but apart from the sanitation, medicine, education, wine, public order, irrigation, roads, the freshwater system and public health, what have the Romans ever done for us?*

Reg, *Monty Python's Life of Brian*, 1979.

* The Romans built sewers and laid plumbing in every territory they conquered. By 344 AD, with over a million people living in Rome, there were more than 140 public toilets.

> "Everybody looks at their poop."

Oprah Winfrey

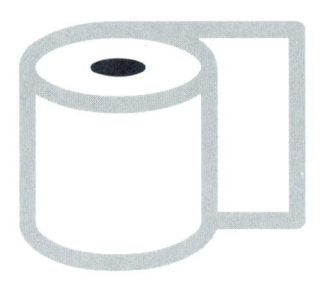

In 1978, Queen Elizabeth II awarded British toilet paper manufacturer Andrex® a Royal Warrant, a prestigious mark of recognition that meant Andrex® was the preferred toilet tissue used in the wiping of royal backsides.

7%

The percentage of Americans who have sent a photo of their feces to a family member or friend, presumably out of concern and/or pride.

EFFLUENCE

A polite term for pooping (if in polite company).

Not the same as affluence.

ONE IN TEN

Americans use a Squatty Potty.*

* For the best pooping position, elevate your knees higher than your hips and keep your feet planted flat. This squatting position helps relax the pelvis and rectum muscles.

BOTTOMS UP

> **Maximum Absorbency Garment (MAG) for Fecal Containment.**

NASA's euphemism for the diapers astronauts used in space.

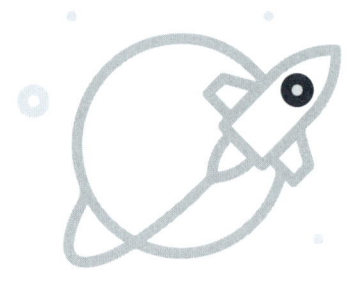

In 2006, President George W. Bush had to poop in a special portable toilet that travelled with him on a trip to Vienna.

It was feared, at the time, that foreign intelligence agencies might seek to collect the President's poop for ransom reasons. (Or, more likely, health issues.)

BOTTOMS UP

> ## We had a fecal fascination in those years.

Tré Cool, Green Day drummer, 2011.

In 1994, American pop-punk band Green Day released the album *Dookie*, a worldwide cultural phenomenon. It sold 20 million copies. The band originally wanted to call the album Liquid Dookie, but the record label said it was too gross. Green Day wanted to name their defining album after diarrhoea in honour of the runs they repeatedly got on tour eating spoiled food.

A TOUCH OF CLOTH

The word "toilet" is derived from the French word *toilette*, which means "dressing room".

The word "toilette" itself has roots derived from another word; *toile*, which means "cloth".

BOTTOMS UP

MONTEZUMA'S REVENGE

Southern and Central American travellers are often cursed by diarrhoea, a condition affectionately known as Montezuma's Revenge.

Montezuma II was the last great Aztec emperor in the 1500s, but his empire was conquered rather emphatically by the Spanish. Aztec legend now states that Montezuma haunts all invaders and looters of his land with his revenge – a severe form of super-poopin'.

Poophephemisms: A–Z

1. Bake a loaf
2. Chop a log
3. Drop the kids off at the pool
4. Float a trout
5. Grow a tail
6. Launch a torpedo
7. Murder a brown snake
8. Pinch a loaf
9. Release the hostage
10. Squeeze the cheese
11. Take the browns to the superbowl
12. Unloose the caboose
13. Visit Boston
14. Wrestle a leprechaun

BOTTOMS UP

> **"**
> I caught my son taking a dump on the upper part of the toilet. He calls it an upper decker.
> **"**

Meredith Palmer, *The Office* (U.S.), Season 6, Episode 6, 2009.

The world's oldest human poop was found at an ancient campfire known as El Salt, Alicante, Spain, in 2014.

Archaeologists believe it to be more than 50,000 years old and to have once belonged to a Neanderthal who had a diet rich in meat and plants.

BOTTOMS UP

> This guy sitting in the row in front of me, Edgar Marsalla, laid this terrific fart. It was a very crude thing to do, in the chapel and all, but it was also quite amusing. Old Marsalla. He damn near blew the roof off.

Holden Caulfield, *The Catcher in the Rye*, J. D. Salinger, 1951.

1935

The year that toilet paper manufacturers were first able to guarantee splinter-free toilet paper.

BOTTOMS UP

> **You can laugh now, but there is an acute shortage of toilet paper.**

Johnny Carson*

* In 1973, Carson cracked a joke about a TP shortage on his *Tonight Show*. There wasn't, but American consumers believed it and went into mass panic mode and bulk bought. Soon there was a shortage – for four months! It got so bad that toilet paper was being sold for big bucks on the black market.

> In my world, everyone's a pony and they all eat rainbows and poop butterflies!

Katie, *Horton Hears a Who!*, 2009.

CHAPTER
FIVE

IT HAPPENS

Pooping is a lot like Fight Club. Everybody loves it, but nobody talks about it. Well, we say, "Forget that!"

We're as serious as a fart attack about poop, as the jokes, quotes, quips and tips in this chapter prove, beyond all rational doubt.

So pull up your sleeves and pull down pants – we're, about to get our hands dirty with even more poop-tastic trivia…

IT HAPPENS

> **There is nothing that will make an Englishman shite so quick as the sight of General Washington.**

Ethan Allen*

* Abraham Lincoln was a huge fan of poop jokes. The above is the punchline to a joke told by Allen that Lincoln loved; he heard that a painting of George Washington had been hung at a British Army outhouse during the War of Independence.

In 2016, Donald Trump asked the Guggenheim Museum to send Vincent van Gogh's "Landscape with Snow" so he could install it in the White House, but the museum refused.

They counteroffered with a functioning solid gold toilet, an artwork by Maurizio Cattelan, entitled "America".

IT HAPPENS

FART ANALYSIS

59% nitrogen

21% hydrogen

9% carbon dioxide

7% methane

4% oxygen

1% hydrogen sulphide
(the guilty party responsible for the stink)

10 FT (6.8 MPH)

The speed of farts per second. The average time it takes for them to sting our nostrils is about 10–15 seconds, depending on the spiciness of the hydrogen sulphide.

IT HAPPENS

SEVEN BILLION

The number of rolls of toilet paper sold in the U.S. each year.

A kitchen sink has 1,250 times more bacteria per square inch than a toilet seat.

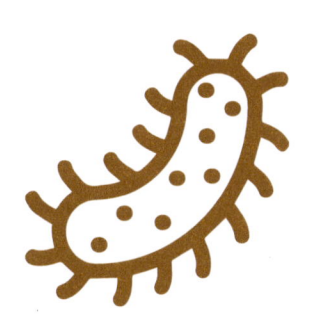

32%

The percentage of men, according to the London School of Hygiene, who wash their hands after using the toilet, compared to 62 per cent of women.

15 MINUTES

The average time an adult American male will spend sitting on the toilet. A female spends, on average, ten minutes less on the toilet.

* We'll let you guess the reason for the time difference.

IT HAPPENS

XYLOSPONGIUM

The word used to describe the non-musical instrument the Ancient Romans wiped their butts with.

It's nothing fancy, just a sponge on a stick… that everyone shared.*

* The phrase "get the wrong end of the stick" originates from these times.

In America's colonial times, when corn was in bountiful supply and founding fathers were signing declarations of independence, a dried-out corn cob doubled as a source of food (first) and an effective butt wiper (second).

IT HAPPENS

Dung beetles love poop.

They'll roll it up in a ball, then roll the ball back to their burrow.

Then a female will lay an egg in the poop, creating both a food source and a first home for their babies.

What a way to live.

O que é um peido para quem está cagado?

What difference does a fart make when you've already shit yourself?

Portuguese proverb (possibly).

IT HAPPENS

The Ancient Greeks wiped their butts with ostraca – a smooth piece of ceramic pottery akin to wiping your bottom with a smooth, round pebble.

What hand do you wipe your butt with?*

* See page 192 for the correct answer.

IT HAPPENS

SCATOMANCY*

Before crystal balls and tarot cards, ancient soothsayers predicted people's fortunes by analysing their poop.

* Different to copromancy, which is how doctors diagnose a person's health based on the shape, size and texture of their poop.

How to Poop at Work

No matter whether it's a line of stalls or a single-use cubicle, pooping at work can be terrifying. Here are five tips to make it less torturous!

1. Carry a notepad, folder or mug around the office – disguise your destination.
2. Make sure the door is locked – there's always one person who checks.
3. Listen to music – drown out the splashes and plops.
4. Flush immediately after pooping – get rid of that smell.
5. Remember you're getting paid to shit.

IT HAPPENS

> **"**
> It is one of those things you would obviously never do when you are not in competition, but I did what I had to do and what was in the rules to win the race. I don't regret it because I won.
> **"**

Paula Radcliffe, London Marathon winner and long-distance running champion.

The world watched in horror when, in 2005, Radcliffe pulled her shorts aside and pooped mid-race live on air. She blamed stomach cramps from bad salmon the night before.

WHY DID THE TOILET PAPER ROLL DOWN THE HILL?

To get to the bottom.

IT HAPPENS

> "
>
> I was in a restaurant in Spain, and I needed to use the facilities. I went to flush. Didn't work. I flushed seven times. Would not work. I found a waiter. He didn't speak English, so I gestured to this man, 'could you come here?' I ushered him into the toilet, I pointed at my poo, I went to flush and it went down straight away. How weird did I look? Like I just invited him into the toilet to say goodbye to my shit.
>
> "

Jack Whitehall on *The Graham Norton Show*, 2019.

1.6 GALLONS

The amount of water required to flush poop.

* Weirdly, this is about the amount of water an average person should drink every day – though not from the toilet.

IT HAPPENS

1857

The year that New Yorker Joseph Gayetty first patented and brought to market your butt's BFF – toilet paper!

* Gayetty didn't call it toilet paper, however. He called it "Medicated Paper for the Water-Closet", which, ironically enough, doesn't have a ring to it.

King Henry VIII, who reigned from 1509–1547, employed manservants known as "Grooms of the Stool", who would attend to the king's toileting needs, including pulling down the oversized monarch's pantaloons and wiping the royal buttocks.

The role continued until 1901, when Edward VII presumably realized he could wipe his own bum.

IT HAPPENS

The first U.S. President, George Washington, had an outhouse at his Mount Vernon, Washington residence.

It had three pooping holes, just one bench and no walls between each hole, suggesting that America's greatest icon liked to poop and party at the same time.

26,500

The amount of poop, in lbs, left by climbers every year at the drop anchor on Mount Everest.

CHAPTER SIX

WIPE OUT

There's no greater feeling in this world than wiping your butt after a perfect poop. We stand by that. And anybody who disagrees needs to eat more fibre.

Before we wipe out for the final time, let's stand up and raise one last toast to poop – life's greatest of guilty pleasures.

For those about to poop, we salute you…

WIPE OUT

> A man may break a word with you, sir; and words are but wind; Ay, and break it in your face, so he break it not behind.

Dromio of Ephesus, *The Comedy of Errors*, William Shakespeare, Act III, Scene I.

> Nicolas let fly a fart as loud as it had been a thunderclap and well-nigh blinded Absolon, poor chap.

Geoffrey Chaucer, *The Canterbury Tales: The Miller's Tale*, 1388.

* One of the first written records of the word fart.

WIPE OUT

In 1722, Jonathan Swift, author of the classic children's tale *Gulliver's Travels*, published *The Benefit of Farting Explained* under the pseudonym Don Fartinando Puff-Indorst, Professor of Bumbast in the University of Crackow.

The book, a celebration of farting says Swift, was "Translated into English at the Request and for the Use of the Lady Damp-Fart of Her-fart-shire by Obadiah Fizzle, Groom of the Stool to the Princess of Arse-Mini in Sardinia."

In 1781, founding Father Benjamin Franklin wrote a humorous essay entitled "Fart Proudly". The essay was a request for scientists to develop a drug that could render farting as "inoffensive" and "as agreeable as perfumes".

"That the permitting this air to escape and mix with the atmosphere, is usually offensive to the company, from the fetid smell that accompanies it. All well-bred people, therefore, to avoid giving such offence, forcibly restrain the efforts of nature to discharge that wind."

WIPE OUT

A wombat's poop is cubed* – not cylindrical – and they poop more than 100 times a day.

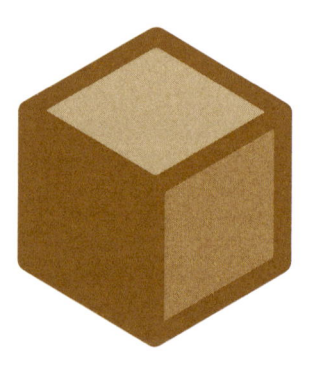

* Cubed poos don't roll off flat surfaces, making them easier to mark the wombat's territories. Now you know!

Adolf Hitler, leader of Germany's Nazi Party during WWII, suffered from severe gastrointestinal cramps for most of his adult life. These cramps resulted in extreme flatulence – fart attacks if you will – that made Hitler's life a misery.

* This isn't a joke, as much as it sounds like one.

WIPE OUT

On 11 September, 2001, an infamous day in modern history, ocean researchers were in the waters of Canada's Bay of Fundy to analyze whale poop. They noticed that the whales' poop showed signs that they were less stressed than usual, a result of the lack of ocean traffic on that day.

The researchers concluded that loud, low-frequency noises from boats cause chronic stress in whales.

12 SECONDS*

The average time it takes mammals, including humans, to poop, as concluded by the Georgia Institute of Technology in a paper titled "The Hydrodynamics of Defecation".

* Your body pushes 0.8 in (2 cm) of poop per second.

WIPE OUT

61.3%

The percentage of Americans who do their daily pooping in the morning.*

* Humans are hardwired to poop predominantly in the morning. This is due to our colons stimulating the release of hormones that trigger contractions in our guts, usually 30 minutes after waking up.

48 HOURS

The approximate time it takes your body to turn digested food in your stomach into poop.

WIPE OUT

Poop Playlist: More Songs to Poop to

1. "Drop It Like It's Hot" – Snoop Dogg
2. "Push It" – Salt-N-Pepa
3. "Free Falling" – Tom Petty
4. "Urgent" – Foreigner
5. "Ring of Fire" – Johnny Cash
6. "Relax" – Frankie Goes to Hollywood
7. "Bat Out of Hell" – Meat Loaf
8. "That Smell" – Lynyrd Skynyrd
9. "Keep Pushin'" – REO Speedwagon
10. "Deuce" – Kiss

4.5 BILLION

The number of people worldwide with no access to a household toilet.*

* According to the United Nations, more than 200 million tons of poop goes untreated every year, sewage that ends up in oceans, lakes and rivers.

WIPE OUT

19 NOVEMBER
WORLD TOILET DAY*

*As officially observed by the United Nations to inspire action to tackle the global sanitation crisis.

1971

The year the first time a toilet was heard flushing on U.S. television. It was for the pilot episode of *All in the Family* on CBS.

WIPE OUT

One person's poop is another person's pleasure.

* While we're here: coprophilia is the term to describe sexual arousal from poop.

Kopi luwak, from Indonesia, is a coffee made from the pooped-out coffee cherries half-digested by the Asian palm civet — a species closely related to weasels. Their poop is collected and turned into rich, steaming and fragrant coffee!

It is the world's most expensive and sought-after coffee.

WIPE OUT

PRURITUS ANI

The term used to describe the strong urge to scratch the skin around your anus after having wiped your butt too much… or too hard… or not enough.

The French word *bidet* (a fancy toilet) is borrowed from the word "pony" (a small horse) due to the straddling position one must adopt when sat above a bidet to wash poop from one's privates.

* According to *Scientific American*, if Americans used bidets instead of toilet paper, 15 million trees could be saved every year.

WIPE OUT

> **Hail Mary, full of grace, the Lord be with me. AAAAHHH!!**

The last lines of Donald Gennaro (Martin Ferrero), who is eaten rather infamously by a Tyrannosaurus rex while sitting on the toilet (and presumably pooping his pants), *Jurassic Park*, 1993.

In Quentin Tarantino's 1993 classic *Pulp Fiction*, Vincent Vega (John Travolta) is seen going to the toilet to poop* three times.

Each time, something bad happens to the character, and ultimately Vega dies in the toilet after being gunned down.

The term "pulp" is a reference to toilet paper.

* Heroin users, like Vega, are constantly constipated.

WIPE OUT

> ## He died fishing his iPhone from a clogged toilet.

Tom Wambsgans (Matthew Macfadyen) about the death of his father-in-law Logan Roy's (played by Brian Cox), who died in the toilet of his private jet, *Succession*, Season 4, Episode 4, 2023.

If you're ever having a shit day, spare a thought for poor pooping Edmund Ironside, King of England in 1016.

He was stabbed in the butthole by a Viking hiding underneath his toilet.

WIPE OUT

> **"**
> # Does the Pope shit in the woods?
> **"**

David Lauren
The Dude, *The Big Lebowski*, 1998.

> By the way, if you're a grown man and you've never shit your pants, you're either a liar, or you're not taking enough chances.

Joe Rogan, 2012.

WIPE OUT

> You know why I get a hotel room? To poop in peace. No kids bangin' on the door, no phones ringin'. It's my time! Every Tuesday and Thursday at 3:00 pm! I don't know why I only go twice a week.

Tracy Jordan, *30 Rock*, Season 3, Episode 22, 2009.

> If aliens are watching us through telescopes, they're going to think the dogs are the leaders of the planet. If you see two life forms, one of them's making a poop, the other one's carrying it for him. Who would you assume is in charge?

Jerry Seinfeld, *Seinfeld*, Season 3, Episode 4, 1991.

WIPE OUT

> 66
>
> The principle, in building a sewer system, was to divert the cause of the mischief to a locality where it can do no mischief.
>
> 99

Sir Joseph William Bazalgette*, 1887.

* The inventor of London's first sewer system in the 1840s, the then-largest in the world.

GHOST WIPE

The term used to describe a poop that leaves no visible trace of its existence on the toilet paper.

WIPE OUT

> **You aren't what you eat — you are what you don't poop.**
>
> **Wavy Gravy**

> If all you do is follow the herd, you'll just be stepping in poop all day.

Wayne Dyer

WIPE OUT

The word "manure" comes from the French "main oeuvre", or "hand work".

* The origins of manure allude to the cultivation of the land by hand. Humans have been fertilizing crops with manure for more than 7,000 years.

New York's
8.5 million residents
produce more than
2.4 million lbs
of poop every day!

WIPE OUT

67%

The percentage of Americans who use their phone while pooping, according to a 2022 survey.

* 27 per cent admitted to taking a phone call mid-poop.

SERIAL POOPERS

Like serial killers, but for poop. Serial poopers are people who brazenly poop in public places, leaving turds in their wake.*

* The opposite of a turd-burglar, a person who pinches poop.

WIPE OUT

If life gives you shit, grow a garden.

In 2019, the UK birthed the world's first ever poo-powered pub, called the Number Two Tavern, in Leeds. The pub employs a ground-breaking process called anaerobic digestion to convert fecal waste into biogas that is used to generate heat and electricity.

WIPE OUT

> **"**
>
> What did they say? Dick Poop. Well, I'm going to change my name to Dick Poop.
>
> **"**

Dick Pope*

* In 2015, Oscars president Cheryl Boone Isaacs mispronounced cinematographer Dick Pope's name during a nomination reading, while standing next to Hollywood heartthrob Chris Penis – sorry, *Pine*.

In 2017, Coloradoan police were on the hunt for a "mad pooper", a jogger who kept pooping outside a family's home every day for weeks on end.

The family saw the pooper once and shouted, "Are you really taking a poop right here in front of my kids?" but the jogger just pooped on.

The pooper is still at large.

WIPE OUT

NOW WASH YOUR HANDS!

* Answer from page 145: The only correct answer is "Toilet paper".